Title

Taking complete Charge of your fertility.

Table of content

Chapter 2

Introduction

Taking Complete Charge of Your Fertility offers everything a potential parent would need to know about the medical and practical hurdles of trying for a child. Fortunately, there are a few regular ways to enhance your fertility. Dietary and lifestyle modifications can help boost fertility

This valuable item answers your questions while providing you with incredible insights into your body.

It covers all aspects of health, from fundamental biology and an explanation of fertility and cycles to describing which supplements are beneficial and which are not, and how you may improve your chances by eating a balanced diet and avoiding alcohol and smoking. There are several tools and guidelines available for parents who are experiencing problems, including a guide to medical alternatives and information on how to obtain more assistance. It will be a great resource for all prospective parents, whether they are starting or expanding their family.

Chapter 1

What factors lead to issues with female fertility?

Female reproductive troubles can be caused by several medical conditions, such as ovulation abnormalities, which impact the ovaries' ability to release eggs. These include thyroid issues (hyperthyroidism or hypothyroidism), hyperprolactinemia, and hormonal abnormalities, including polycystic ovarian syndrome. Polyps or fibroids in the uterus are examples of uterine or cervical abnormalities. Pelvic inflammatory illness is a common cause of fallopian tube damage or obstruction. When tissue that typically lines the lining of the uterus develops outside of it, it can result in endometriosis. When the ovaries cease functioning and menstruation ends before the age of forty, this condition is known as primary ovarian insufficiency or early menopause.

Pelvic adhesions are bands of scar tissue that form following abdominal or pelvic surgery, appendicitis, or pelvic infection. illnesses, including poorly managed diabetes, celiac disease, and some autoimmune disorders like lupus that are linked to not having menstruation. Age is another factor. It's possible that delaying pregnancy will make it less likely that you'll get pregnant. It becomes more difficult to conceive as you age since your eggs' number and quality decrease. maximizing the likelihood of becoming pregnant. Recognize when to ovulate. Only having intercourse on the day of ovulation or during the five days preceding it makes pregnancy probable. We refer to this as the fruitful window. Your best chance of becoming pregnant is to conceive during the fertile window, namely the three days preceding and including ovulation.

how can you tell whether you are ovulating?

The duration of your menstrual cycle determines this. If your cycle lasts 28 days on average, then day one is the first day of your period, and you ovulate on day 14. This occurs around 14 days before the commencement of your menstruation. This indicates that days 12, 13, and 14 are the most fertile for you to have intercourse. Your most fruitful days for sex are days 19, 20, and 21, and ovulation occurs around day 21 if your menstrual cycle is 35 days on average. In the event that your cycle is shorter let's say 21 days ovulation occurs approximately on day seven, and days five, six, and seven are the most fertile. This ovulation calculator will assist you in determining your C window. Your chances of becoming pregnant should increase if you have intercourse every two to three days if your cycle is erratic and if you are unable to determine when you ovulate.

The fundamental: It seems like your health instructor in high school told you that you may become pregnant at any time you had sex. However, the reality is a little more nuanced. Your body goes through a series of hormonal changes every month that lead to the growth and maturation of an immature egg in the ovary. Every menstrual cycle is unique. Starting with the last menstrual cycle, the last phases of egg development and ovulation take around two weeks on average.

Ovulation

Ovulation is the process by which an egg is expelled from the ovary once it has reached maturity. After that, the egg moves toward the uterus via the fallopian tube. Once released, the egg is only viable for around twenty-four hours. The fertilized egg often continues on its path into the uterus if a sperm cell fertilizes the egg during this window of time. After that, it usually implants into the lining of the uterus. Having intercourse in the days preceding and during ovulation is crucial. In this manner, when the egg is delivered, the sperm cells are in the fallopian tubes. Fertilization can happen more easily as a result. Up to five days are allowed for sperm to survive in the female reproductive system.

Choosing the appropriate time and making sure that your intercourse is occurring at the appropriate point in your cycle is the best strategy to improve your chances of becoming pregnant rapidly. In the event that your cycles are regular, you should ovulate around two weeks before your period.

your window of opportunity for conception will probably be around five days before your anticipated ovulation and one day following. The closer you get to ovulation, the higher the likelihood. It might be a little trickier to anticipate when you will ovulate and what your viable window will be if you have irregular periods. You may utilize a variety of methods to help determine your ovulation and viable window more precisely.

Kits for predicting ovulation: These kits resemble pregnancy tests that are done with urine. A few days before, when you anticipate your period, you will start peeing on the test strips once or twice a day. Luteinizing hormone (LH), which spikes just prior to ovulation, is detected by the test strips. If your test results are positive (see your instructions for specifics), you should have intercourse that day and the next day. After that, fertility usually declines dramatically.

Normal body temperature.

If you take your basal body temperature (BBT) three times in a row before getting out of bed, you may be able to see a very little drop in temperature followed by a very slight rise in temperature. The increase in temperature might be as minor as 0.5°C. This may indicate that ovulation has occurred. Remember that an egg only lasts for around 24 hours following **ovulation**, so this supposed "fertile window" might not be a reliable guide for when you should engage in sexual activity. A shift in BBT suggests that you could have missed the window since after ovulation has happened, there is a very low likelihood of conception, and a rise in BBT is an indication that ovulation has occurred. All of this indicates that if you're attempting to get pregnant, BBT is not a trustworthy way to schedule sexual activity. There are further worries that this procedure isn't always accurate due to several reasons that might raise body temperature, such as illness. It might be challenging for some ladies to notice that temperature increases.

Vaginal mucus variations:

Your estrogen level increases when the ovarian follicle, a little sac in the ovary that houses the developing egg, grows. The thin, slick cervical mucus is a result of this estrogen surge. Additionally, you can observe a rise in cervical mucus. You should start having sex every day or every other day until ovulation as soon as you see these changes. Your cervical mucus will thicken and become sticky after ovulation. It could also seem hazy. Follicle observation: You can discuss your alternatives with your doctor if the aforementioned techniques aren't working for you while tracking your ovulation. Some physicians will check you with routine ovulation ultrasounds and blood hormone checks. This will enable you to confirm if you are ovulating or to determine the precise time of your ovulation.

A miscarriage is what?

When a baby or embryo leaves the uterus before 20 weeks of gestation, it is called a miscarriage. Often, severe bleeding, followed by cramps and back or stomach discomfort, is the first indication that something is happening. These symptoms may continue for as little as a few days, similar to a regular period, or for as long as three or four weeks, depending on how far along your pregnancy was. Consult your physician as soon as possible if you encounter any of these signs.

What follows a miscarriage?
Your doctor will use an ultrasound to confirm the miscarriage and may also examine your cervix during a pelvic exam. In order to assess blood loss, check your hCG levels, and check for Rh incompatibility, he or she may also take a blood sample. You could also be given an injection of Rh immunoglobulin if your Rh factor is Rh-negative to avoid major complications in subsequent pregnancies. removing the uterus Your uterus must be empty after the miscarriage is diagnosed in order for your regular menstrual cycle to

continue and, if desired, for you to attempt pregnancy once more. It's conceivable that the miscarriage was "complete," that all of the baby tissue had already been removed from your uterus, if your first indication of a miscarriage was severe bleeding, particularly if it happened soon after you became pregnant. However, occasionally a miscarriage isn't complete, and pieces of the pregnancy remain in the uterus (known as an incomplete miscarriage) that need to be removed. This is most common the later in the first trimester you are. This can occur in a variety of ways, including.

anticipatory supervision.

You might decide to wait for the pregnancy meaningto end naturally and let nature take its course. It might take a few days or, in some circumstances, three or four weeks to wait it out after a missed or partial miscarriage before your body heals and your monthly cycles return to normal

Drugs

. Your doctor may alternatively offer you the option to take miscarriage drugs, often misoprostol or misoprostol plus mifepristone, to hasten the process if there are no signs of your body removing the embryo on its own. After taking a pill or getting a vaginal suppository, you should begin to bleed and pass placental and fetal tissue within a few hours.

Each woman experiences this differently, but most will pass the tissue in a day or two. Some of the negative effects of these treatments are similar to what you may have experienced if you had just allowed nature to take its course, such as diarrhea, cramps, bleeding, and nausea.

surgery.

Dilation and curettage (D&C), a small procedure, is an additional alternative. A specialist will carefully remove the placental and fetal tissue from your uterus during this surgery. Within the operation, bleeding normally stops within a week or so. After a D&C, there is a small chance of infection, even though adverse effects are uncommon. How is severe cramping and bleeding, the miscarriage is most likely far advanced. If so, it would be better to let it develop organically rather than doing a D&C. However, misoprostol or a D&C can be preferable options if there is no bleeding (as in the case of a missed miscarriage). Your physical and mental condition. For a woman and her partner, if she has one, waiting for a natural miscarriage to happen after a fetus has passed away in gestation can be very taxing. You probably won't be able to start mourning or come to grips with your loss while you're still pregnant. When and if the time is perfect, you can try to conceive again, and you can restart your menstrual periods sooner if the procedure is completed more quickly. advantages and risks. A D&C has a very modest (but still extremely minimal) risk of infection due to its intrusive nature. For most women, however, the advantages of suffering a miscarriage sooner may well exceed that little risk. There's a chance that a naturally occurring miscarriage won't empty the uterus entirely, in which case a D&C could be required to complete what nature has begun. An assessment of the stillbirth. It will be simpler to determine the reason for the miscarriage by looking at the fetal tissue after a D&C.

Not sure what to do following a miscarriage?

Regardless of whether you underwent surgery to manage your miscarriage, your doctor will advise you on whether it's safe to get back to your regular routine, which includes **exercise and sexual activity.**

Your doctor may advise you to resume your regular activities immediately after the procedure, but in order to prevent infection, it is advised that you refrain from sexual activity and the use of tampons for a period of two weeks. A few weeks following your loss, make sure to schedule a follow-up visit with your healthcare physician. What to be aware of following a miscarriage: Your doctor will probably want to follow up with you for a few weeks or months after your miscarriage, even if everything goes smoothly and without any discomfort (don't worry, they are all extremely unusual). If your bleeding persists for more than seven days, it may indicate an infection or that placental tissue is still present in your uterus.

Abdominal discomfort, fever, chills, and foul-smelling discharge are some other indicators of an infection. Your doctor will probably prescribe an antibiotic course if they detect an illness. Retained products of conception, the official word for any embryo, fetal, or placental tissue left in your uterus, can very rarely begin to grow abnormally and develop into a kind of tumor known as a choriocarcinoma. You also run a small chance of experiencing surgical complications following a D&C. About 16 percent of women who have their first D&C experience Asherman syndrome, a scarring condition that occurs inside the uterus or around the cervix. Fortunately, you'll heal and be able to conceive once more. However, it could require a second procedure to remove those scars.

Your post-miscarriage feelings:

The stages of mourning You may probably feel a wide range of emotions and reactions after losing a pregnancy. Understanding them will eventually help you accept your loss, even though you can't wish them away. Many people go through several stages on their path to emotional healing after experiencing a loss of any kind. These phases are typical, although the sensations you experience and the sequence in which the first three occur are also subject to change. Disbelief and shock. The idea that "this couldn't have happened to me" may accompany feelings of numbness and disbelief. This is a psychological defense mechanism used to shield your mind from the anguish of loss. guilt and fury. You could blame yourself, thinking that you must have done something wrong to cause the miscarriage or that the baby would still be alive if you had been happier during the pregnancy, in an attempt to place the blame for such a senseless tragedy. Alternatively, even if there's no justification, you can hold God or your practitioner responsible for allowing this to occur. When someone close to you becomes a parent or becomes pregnant, you could feel jealous, resentful, and even briefly hostile toward them. dejection and hopelessness. You could cry all the time, feel depressed most of the time, or find it difficult to eat or sleep. Along with losing all interest in life and being unable to do anything else, you might also be wondering if you'll ever be able to have a healthy child.

Acceptance.

You will eventually accept the loss. Remember that this only indicates that you will be able to accept the loss and return to your daily activities, not that you will forget it. Assistance for miscarriages: You may have intense feelings of loss, regardless of how early in your pregnancy you experienced the death of a baby. The sadness you are experiencing is real. Some well-meaning friends and family members might attempt to downplay the significance by saying, "Don't worry, you can try again," but they are unaware of how traumatic losing a baby can be at any point during a pregnancy. Nevertheless, it's critical to keep in mind that you are entitled to mourn as much or as little as necessary, whether you have experienced a miscarriage, an ectopic pregnancy, or a molar pregnancy. Use this as a means to aid in your healing and eventual transition. If you have a partner, turn to them for assistance.

Recall that although he or she may express their grief differently, they are also grieving the death of a baby. You can both heal if you communicate your feelings honestly to one another rather than attempting to shield one another. Seek advice from your pastor, priest, rabbi, or other spiritual leader if you're religious. Maybe a private ceremony, just you and your spouse, or with close family members, may provide you with closure. It may also be comforting to express your thoughts to other women who have had miscarriages, whether it be online, with a friend, or in a support group.

To assist you through this trying time, ask your practitioner for a recommendation for a therapist or grief support group. As a result of the high rate of miscarriages among women (between 10 and 20 percent of pregnancies terminate in miscarriage), you might be shocked to learn how many people you know have experienced the same thing but have never discussed it with you or perhaps never discussed it at all. Don't share your sentiments if you don't feel like it or if you don't think you should. Just do what is best for you.

When will you feel back to normal?

Give yourself time, regardless of how you're feeling, which might be all over the place considering your current circumstances. Recognize that you could always have feelings of sadness or melancholy for the pregnancy you lost and that even years after the miscarriage, you might still experience these emotions on the anniversary of the due date of your lost child. If it helps, schedule a particular activity that will be upbeat and help you recall it at that time. This could be planting a tree or some fresh flowers, going on a peaceful picnic in the park, or having a nice meal with your significant other. At least for the first year or two. You should start to feel better with time, even though it's appropriate to grieve your loss and vital to process it in your manner. Professional counseling can assist you in recovering if you don't if you're still having problems adjusting to daily life (you're not sleeping or eating, you're not able to concentrate at work, you're isolating yourself from family and friends), or if you're still experiencing extreme anxiety (research has shown that anxiety after miscarriage is even more common than depression).

Resuming pregnancy following a miscarriage:

It used to be recommended by medical professionals to wait many months following a miscarriage before attempting to become pregnant again. However, they have discovered that the uterus is incredibly adept at healing following a miscarriage. Nowadays, the majority of physicians advise trying again as soon as you've experienced one regular menstrual period. However, discuss your unique circumstances with your practitioner. He or she may suggest a longer delay if there is scarring in your uterus or if placenta fragments were left behind. About 65 to 75 percent of women who have experienced two or three unplanned pregnancy losses in a row go on to have a successful subsequent pregnancy that results in a live delivery. Remind yourself that you are capable of becoming pregnant again and that you will probably give birth to a healthy child. The majority of women view miscarriages as one-time occurrences and even as predictors of future fertility.

Advantages of recording your cycle:

You may become an expert on your health and an advocate for your well-being by learning about your menstrual cycle and getting to know your body. Using an app, a fertility awareness chart, or a menstrual calendar may all be beneficial to you. Although there are several "schools" and variations of them, there are two fundamental methods. Although they are distinct, menstrual cycle awareness and fertility awareness can be combined to increase menstrual self-knowledge even further. You can use a print or online diary or calendar to record when you bleed, whether or not you have vaginal secretions, and whether or not you experience any of the following physical or emotional changes: pain or cramping, heavier or lighter flow, changes in mood, energy level, or sexual desire, swollen or tender breasts, breakouts on your skin, or any changes in your overall physical or mental health. Menstrual charts and period tracking applications are readily available on the internet.

Advantages of Charting your period

Charting allows us to see changes in mood, energy, or health connected to cycles that we would only be able to speculate about if we didn't keep a record. There may be periods during your cycle when you're usually energized or depleted; sexy or uncomfortable being touched; outgoing or reserved; nervous, furious, or calm. Knowing your cyclical tendencies will help you make plans to benefit from life's volatility. For a period at least, keeping a monthly cycle journal may put you in better physical and mental alignment. Understanding your cycles can also help you make sense of changes in your body and emotions that might otherwise seem random. Menstrual cycle tracking is a useful tool for monitoring and evaluating our gynecological health. Are our cycles regular, lasting around the same amount of time each time? How severe is our monthly pain, and how long does it last? How much do we bleed, and how many menstrual cups, pads, or tampons do we use? Do we experience emotional shifts in sync with our cycles? Our charts can offer us useful information to learn from and provide to our healthcare doctors if we have any concerns about gynecological issues. Charting can assist us in tracking the duration of our menstrual cycle, the onset and duration of its onset, the occurrence of excessive bleeding, and any symptoms we may be experiencing throughout the perimenopause, the period of time before our periods end permanently. Understanding this information can greatly benefit our understanding of the perimenopausal period. Seeing a healthcare professional might also be beneficial in helping us manage our symptoms. Knowing the workings of your reproductive system. Recognize Your Monthly Routine Understanding your menstrual cycle increases your likelihood of becoming pregnant. The first day of your menstrual flow marks the beginning of the first phase.

Maximizing pregnancy occurance (your hormones)

Follicle-stimulating hormone (FSH), among other hormones, is released by your body to cause the eggs in your ovaries to develop. These hormones also aid in thickening your uterine lining between days two and fourteen, preparing it for a fertilized egg. We refer to this as the follicular stage. The Events Involved in Ovulation The menstrual cycle lasts 28 to 35 days on average. Typically, ovulation takes place between days 11 and 21 of your cycle. The most mature egg is released when luteinizing hormone (LH), a hormone, rises. Your cervical mucus also gets more slick to aid sperm in reaching the egg at the same time. Everything Relies on Timing: Only 300 to 400 of the 1 million–2 million eggs that women have at birth are released over their lifetimes during ovulation. You usually only release one every month. One of the two fallopian tubes that connect your ovaries to your uterus is where the egg travels. On its trip to the uterus, sperm may fertilize it if the time is right. The egg dissolves if fertilization does not occur within 24 hours of the egg exiting the ovary. Knowing when you are ovulating might help you and your partner schedule sex for when you are most likely to get pregnant because sperm only survive for three to five days. Keep a Record of Your Most Fruitful Days. Generally speaking, having intercourse 1-2 days prior to ovulation increases the likelihood of getting pregnant. If your cycle is typically 28 days, then subtract 14 days from the anticipated start of your next period. Around that time, aim to have sex every other day, say on days 12 and 14. You may determine the most likely day by using an online ovulation calculator or over-the-counter ovulation and depending on how long or short your cycle is. Hormone-Based Ovulation Prediction: Your ovaries release an egg in response to an increase in LH. The spike often occurs thirty-six hours prior to the discharge of the egg. LH levels and other hormones are measured by ovulation and fertility monitoring kits to assist in determining the day of ovulation. These kits are very accurate, extremely portable, and employ hormones. They also come in wearable form.

To see the increase in LH, you might choose to test one or two days before when you anticipate the spike. The Final Stage of Your Monthly Routine: Progesterone helps prime the lining of your uterus for a fertilized egg by acting throughout the second part of your menstrual cycle. In the event that the egg is not fertilized and does not implant, it disintegrates, progesterone levels drop, and after 12 to 16 days, the egg is expelled from the body along with blood and uterine lining tissues. It is the menstrual cycle. Usually, it lasts three to seven days.

Chapter 2

In contrast to males, who are constantly producing sperm, women have all the egg cells they will ever have at birth, and as they age, this quantity gradually decreases. Your remaining eggs will also become lower quality, which raises the possibility of infertility and loss.

The quantity of eggs you have is unchangeable, but the quality of the eggs is.

The road toward conception in the complex realm of fertility is significantly influenced by the quality of a woman's eggs. We will examine foods that may improve egg quality, a crucial factor that frequently coexists with successful conception, in our investigation of nutrition's influence on female reproductive health. Together, we will explore the science

Underlying egg health as well as useful nutritional and lifestyle recommendations.

Our goal is to provide women with the information they need to nurture their eggs using the abundance of nature.

Comprehending the Quality of Female Eggs

Egg Quality: What Is It?

Despite its seeming elusiveness, egg quality is a crucial component of fertility. It speaks to the DNA integrity of an egg and its ability to effectively fertilize. Egg quality is influenced by a multitude of factors, including age, genetics, and lifestyle choices. Age and genetics cannot be changed, but lifestyle decisions including food can be made to promote the healthiest possible eggs.

The Relationship Between Egg Quality and Nutrition

The effects of our diets go much beyond just pleasing our palates; they affect our reproductive health at its most fundamental level. Our food is a quiet architect, sculpting complex hormone balance, fostering the delicate dance of cellular functions, and even strengthening our defenses against the unseen threat of oxidative stress. Every nutrient is a keynote in a symphony that perfectly orchestrates the smooth operation of our reproductive systems.

Think of nutrition as the strings that create the melodic hum of hormonal homeostasis, and the body as a well-tuned instrument. Our diet's vitamins, minerals, and antioxidants serve as the building blocks that create an atmosphere that is conducive to conception. By affecting our eggs' DNA, these nutritional architects create the framework for robust cellular foundations.

The amazing thing about it all is that we are the ones with the paintbrush, using careful nutritional selections to create this canvas of reproductive well-being. The veggies we select, the healthy grains we eat, and the omega-3-rich seafood we enjoy are all parts of a complex picture that may improve the quality of our eggs. Therefore, every mouthful we take reminds us that the decisions we make now can have a positive impact in the future and that our choices have an impact on our reproductive journey.

Components that Improve the Quality of Eggs

Antioxidants: Protectors of the Health of Eggs

Nature's defense against oxidative stress, which can harm cells and lower the quality of eggs, is antioxidants. Antioxidants are abundant in leafy greens, which are loaded with vitamins A and E, and berries, which are high in anthocyanins and vitamin C. Nuts like walnuts and almonds also include a good amount of vitamin E and selenium, which are both necessary for protecting eggs from oxidative damage

Omega-3 Fatty Acids: Encouraging Hormone Homeostasis
The anti-inflammatory and hormone-regulatory qualities of omega-3 fatty acids are well known. Including plant-based foods like walnuts and flaxseeds, as well as fatty fish like trout and salmon, in your diet can help to create a balanced hormonal environment that promotes good egg development.

Folate: Essential to the Integrity of DNA

One of the essential B vitamins for DNA synthesis and repair is folate. It is crucial to make sure you are getting enough folate, especially in the early stages of pregnancy and before conception. Lentils, avocados, and dark leafy greens are great sources of folate that help preserve the genetic integrity of your egg.

Vitamin D: Strengthening the Reproductive System

Vitamin D, sometimes called the "sunshine vitamin," affects menstrual cycles and hormone levels, which in turn affect reproductive health. Egg health can be promoted by exposure to sunshine and consumption of foods high in vitamin D, such as fortified dairy products, fatty fish, and egg yolks.

Filling the reproductive system with oxygen

Iron is a reproductive health hero who goes unnoticed. It guarantees that tissues including those found in the reproductive organs are properly oxygenated. Egg health may be promoted by a rich iron supply found in red meat, beans, and spinach, which can help to maintain healthy blood flow.

B vitamins: vitality and quality of eggs

B vitamins, including B6 and B12, are essential for cellular activity and energy metabolism. B vitamins are essential for maintaining energy levels and promoting the formation of healthy eggs. A balanced diet rich in whole grains, lean meats, and leafy greens delivers an abundance of these nutrients.

Plant-Based Diets for Healthy Eggs

Foods High in Phytoestrogen: Achieving Hormonal Balance

Phytoestrogens are interesting partners in the intricate hormonal ballet that controls our reproductive system. These organic substances, which may be found in some plant-based diets, have the amazing capacity to replicate the actions of estrogen in our bodies. They provide a mild prod to our complex endocrine system; therefore, their importance in maintaining hormonal equilibrium cannot be overstated. Legumes, flaxseeds, and soy products are important components of phytoestrogen-rich diets. By adding these foods to our diet, we may be creating an atmosphere in which our hormones oscillate in a rhythmic pattern, which may help preserve the balance of reproduction.

Fruits to Enhance the Quality of Female Eggs

Vibrant Fruits and Vegetables: The Natural Antioxidant Powerhouse

Vibrant fruits and vegetables not only conjure up visual feasts for the eyes, but they also open the door to a wealth of antioxidants that nature has so kindly supplied. In the fight against oxidative stress, a persistent force that might jeopardize our reproductive health, these antioxidants are devoted warriors. The vitamins and phytonutrients hidden in the rainbow of hues are powerful friends in this battle. These nutrients have the amazing ability to potentially improve the quality of eggs by reducing cellular damage and inflammation. By consuming juicy berries and crisp kale leaves, we are providing our bodies with natural defenses against the sneaky attacker known as oxidative stress.

Avocados: Avocados are a good choice for a fruit that is high in nutrients. It will assist you in maintaining good reproductive health and enhancing the quality of your eggs due to its high monounsaturated fat content.

Nuts and dried fruit: Nuts and dried fruit are an excellent source of vitamins, minerals, protein, and antioxidants. Brazil nuts have a high selenium content. This mineral serves as a barrier against dangerous chemicals and aids in the protection of eggs from injury. This contributes even more to improved egg production.

Berries: Rich in vitamin C, folate (also known as folic acid), and potent antioxidants, berries are a superfood. They support the health and strength of eggs in addition to protecting them from dangerous free radicals.

Items to steer clear of, for improved chance of pregnancy.

Being aware of what you put in your mouth is crucial while attempting to increase your chances of getting pregnant. Due to their inflammatory properties, which are linked to reproductive problems including endometriosis and PCOS, some foods may interfere with your goals.

Soy: Reducing your soy consumption is a wise idea. Despite all of soy's advantages, it also contains substances that are quite similar to estrogen. Consuming too much soy, particularly in processed forms like bars and powders, can throw off your hormone balance. A soy diet high in estrogen may affect your ability to conceive.

Alcohol: You may want to limit your alcohol intake while you try to get pregnant. Regular drinking has been linked to decreased fertility and more difficult conception, according to research. Additionally, it is a wonderful time to give up smoking. Cigarette nicotine is not good for eggs.

Refined sugars: such as high-fructose corn syrup, should be avoided. They might cause your blood sugar to fluctuate erratically when consumed in excess. These variations may cause issues for your reproductive system. Consuming too much sugar can also upset your hormonal and insulin balance, which may make getting pregnant more challenging.

Stay away from all trans fats.

Steer clear of trans fats at all costs, as they can promote insulin resistance and complicate your body's use of glucose. This may make conception difficult in addition to disrupting your ovulation cycle. Evidence from studies indicates that eating more trans fats increases your likelihood of developing reproductive issues connected to ovulation.

Where may these trans fats be found?

In a lot of snack bags and store-bought baked goods

Certain foods are derived from animals.

Popular dishes such as french fries

Some varieties of margarine

Consequently, if you want to become pregnant soon, be sure to stay away from the foods listed above.

Steer clear of overly processed carbs.

Aim to increase the amount of complex or slow-digesting carbohydrates in your diet by including whole grains, legumes, fruits, vegetables, and brown rice. These healthy, high-fiber carbohydrates gradually control your insulin and blood sugar levels. However, because highly processed carbohydrates readily transform into sugar, avoiding them is also imperative.

Animal Sources of Proteins: When you're attempting to conceive, proteins from animals such as fish, meat, and eggs also come into play. For example, eating sardines and salmon is good for aspiring moms and is safe. They include essential nutrients that aid in the development of the baby's neurological system, such as omega-3 fatty acids and DHA. Another form of protein is eggs, which are also a great source of choline and omega 3, two nutrients that are vital for a developing baby's brain. For optimum nourishment, doctors frequently recommend organic eggs.

The significance of egg quality in conception

The journey to parenthood is significantly influenced by the quality of the eggs. Throughout the 90-day maturation period, several factors, like nutrition, stress, lifestyle, and general health, affect the quality of the eggs.

Good-quality eggs entail:

The chances of sperm fertilizing the egg are higher.

Increased likelihood that the embryo will implant in the uterus. Egg quality may be influenced by age, and as women age, fewer and lower-quality eggs are produced. Therefore, although women in their 30s and 40s can still become pregnant, they may require more medical assistance or should take extra care of their health, which includes consuming a nutritious diet.

What indicates poor egg quality?

Here are several indicators that your eggs may not be at their best:

- Having difficulties becoming pregnant
- Periods that arrive late or don't arrive every month
- Periods that are shorter than normal

To find out if the quality of your eggs is acceptable, you can do various tests. The anti-mullerian hormone (AMH) blood test is often used by many people to monitor their egg supply. Another method to find out about your egg reserve is to undergo a specialized ultrasound. Doctors count the follicles, which are tiny sacs found in your ovaries, during this examination. Your doctor will calculate your antral follicle count by adding these follicles together. This can help you estimate the number of eggs remaining in your ovaries.

Vitamins to increase the chances of conception

What is known, though, is that vitamins are vital to every process in our bodies, including reproduction. Vitamins are utilized in

•   Women's ovulation and menstruation

• Function of the thyroid

• Production of energy

• The immune system

• Egg maturation and quality

Supplementing with specific vitamins might be beneficial if we are lacking in them, and in certain situations, it can help lessen the symptoms of infertility, such as polycystic ovarian syndrome (PCOS). Not just women should think about using fertility medications; several supplements have also been proven to improve sperm motility and quality.

Please remember that using supplements should never take the place of a well-balanced diet; instead, we should constantly strive to obtain as many vitamins, minerals, and other nutrients as possible through a healthy diet.

1.   Coenzyme Q10

Benefits for women: Coenzyme Q10 may enhance the ovarian response to in vitro fertilization.

Benefits for males include increased sperm motility.

Naturally occurring in our bodies, coenzyme Q10 aids in the creation of energy inside our cells. Regrettably, as we age, our bodies produce less of this enzyme. Re-raising it using a supplement may improve fertility, particularly in the case of IVF.

Dosage: The suggested dosage varies according to your individual needs; however, it may be as little as 200 mg for males and 300–1000 mg for women each day.

2.   Acetyl L-carnitine

Benefits for women: The antioxidants included in acetyl L-carnitine support a healthy female reproductive system.

Benefits for men: improves the motility of sperm

Acetyl L-carnitine (ALC) is a naturally occurring derivative of the amino acid L-carnitine (LC), which aids in the conversion of fat into energy. It is believed to help slow down the reproductive system's aging process.

Compared to LC, acetyl L-carnitine has more potent antioxidant qualities that are especially beneficial for female fertility. However, PCOS, endometriosis, and the lack of menstruation (amenorrhea) can all benefit from taking both (ALC) and (LC) together.

Dose: For both genders, 1-3g per day is the recommended range.

3. Vitamin E

Benefits for women: In general, vitamin E can support healthy endometrial growth and improve the health of female reproduction.

Benefits for males include increased sperm motility.

The antioxidant vitamin E has the ability to improve male and female fertility. Infertility in both sexes has been connected to low vitamin E levels.

Dosage: 15 milligrams daily.

4.Omega-3s

Benefits for women: Women over the age of 35 may benefit most from omega-3 fatty acids.

Benefits for men: it can raise the general caliber of sperm.

Essential to human health, omega-3 fatty acids have been associated with better implantation of embryos, a reduction in preterm labor, and enhanced sperm motility, morphology, and quantity.

Dosage: It's best to attempt to obtain these from a balanced diet that includes foods like nuts and fatty fish.

5. Mineral Selenium

Benefits for women: Research suggests that selenium may lower the chance of miscarriage.

Benefits for men: it can also raise the general caliber of sperm.

The strong mineral selenium is crucial to the body's operation and has a special significance for the reproductive system. It may also support the development of strong follicles in the ovaries.

Low semen quality and motility, as well as miscarriages, have been related to deficiencies in selenium.

50 mcg daily is the dose.

Avoiding pollutants in the environment

There are some little-known environmental exposures that can subtly impair both men's and women's ability to conceive, which can either increase or decrease fertility.

There are poisons found in the environment, both naturally and through chemicals. It may surprise you to learn that pregnant women are thought to be exposed to a minimum of forty-three toxins. These substances have the ability to pass through the placenta and cause illness and exposure in fetuses.

Reducing exposure can improve a woman's chances of getting pregnant and maintain the health of both mother and child. I want to walk you through the four main offenders and how to avoid them.

Fertility may be harmed by

- **Heavy metals.**

Fertility can be severely impacted by heavy metals, including cadmium, lead, and mercury.

Preconception exposure to lead, mercury, and cadmium: does it impact the success of infertility treatments? The researchers discovered a correlation between lower rates of embryo implantation and egg fertilization and elevated cadmium levels.

Face lotions and mercury thermometers contain mercury, a neurotoxin that has been connected to low IQ, poor language and motor development, and other issues. Fish including king mackerel, shark, swordfish, marlin, orange roughy, and bigeye tuna are known to have high mercury levels since mercury may also leak into the ocean as an industrial byproduct. When trying to conceive, women should restrict their intake of these fish and avoid them if they are pregnant or nursing. Nevertheless, fish is a valuable source of omega-3 fatty acids, protein, and healthy fats. Try to have one or two meals of mercury-free seafood per week, including shrimp and salmon.

- **Lead:**

is present in older homes and in those who renovate older homes. It's also present in jewelry, imported ceramics, traditional medicines, and pica. In addition to being neurotoxic, lead has been linked to miscarriage and hypertension during pregnancy. Rechargeable batteries, plastic manufacturing, organ meats, paint pigment, cigarette smoke, and insecticides all contain cadmium. Increased levels can cause low birth weight, smaller heads, and mental problems in boys.

- **Cadmium**

has been connected to lower testosterone levels, motility, and sperm quality in males. Cadmium can cause irregular menstrual periods in women.

Steer clear of exposure sources whenever you can. If you're not sure, be tested for exposure to lead, cadmium, or mercury.

Pesticides affect a mother's and her child's health.

According to estimates, 90% of people have pesticide levels in their blood and urine that may be detected. In the environment, pesticides can linger, gradually deteriorating and polluting our food, water, air, dust, and soil. Antenatal and perinatal pesticide exposure can affect the health of both the mother and the fetus. Reduced intrauterine growth, miscarriage, low birth weight, poor IQ, and an increased incidence of leukemia and testicular cancer in children have all been associated with it.

Pesticides and insecticides should be kept out of the house and away from pets. Agricultural workers should remove their shoes before entering a residence, wear the proper protective gear, and wash their hands after work. When choosing fruit, it's crucial to be organic, especially when it comes to the Dirty Dozen grapes, plums, peaches, string beans, potatoes, kale, strawberries, apples, pears, vegetables, celery, and peppers.

BPA and other endocrine disruptors can affect the quality of eggs.

Chemicals known to alter hormone synthesis can affect the results of reproduction. Polybrominated diethyl ethers (PBDEs), phthalates, and bisphenol A (BPA) are the three primary compounds that are of concern.

Plastics, metal can liners, cash register receipts, laptops, mobile phones, and reusable food containers are all known to contain BPA. Exposure to BPA can happen by eating, drinking, or absorbing it through the skin. BPA has been shown to have deleterious effects on placenta development, rates of genetic normalcy, egg quality, and embryonic development. Due to BPA concerns, "BPA-free" plastics which frequently include bisphenol S, an equally hazardous substance have become popular. Limit the use of plastic containers, especially while reheating food in microwaves, and replace them with glass and stainless steel containers instead of plastic ones in order to prevent harmful toxins. Steer clear of thermal paper receipts from cash registers, canned goods, and water bottles with the numbers 3 or 7 written on the bottom.

Phthalates are man-made chemicals that are present in floor processors, toys, IV tubing, food processing, and body lotions. According to a study examining the effects of environmental exposures on IVF results, phthalates may decrease the number of retrieved eggs and the rate of conception, but they also raise the risk of preterm delivery and pregnancy loss before 20 weeks. There is a correlation between exposure and increased sperm DNA damage in males. For cooking and drinking, switch to glass or steel instead of plastic; furthermore, cut back on heating meals in plastic and reduce the amount of prepared or quick food.

PBDEs are flame retardants found in electronics, carpets, fabrics, and upholstered furniture. These days, flame-retardant substitutes mostly replace them in the United States. They have a half-life of up to 12 years, which is terrible news. Pregnancy exposure to flame retardants has been connected to anomalies in the mother's thyroid, especially in California, where they are used more often. According to other research, 28% of individuals with higher preconceptional PBDE levels also had a greater prevalence of pregnancy loss. In the same vein, greater levels in kids throughout the neurodevelopment stage have been connected to kids' lower IQs or lack of focus. If there is any exposure, remove your shoes and wash your hands before entering the house. Make sure the furniture is free of PBDEs before you buy it, and keep kids away from freshly upholstered furniture that has PBDEs.

Pregnancy can have negative effects from air pollution.

Research has indicated a connection between air pollution and unfavorable pregnancy outcomes such as low birth weight, premature delivery, stillbirth, and early pregnancy loss. The results of the study link air pollution to reduced IQ in children and miscarriages. Research examining the effects of living close to a roadway also revealed increased infertility rates. Use HEPA filters inside your home and stay indoors during periods of low air quality, even when it is hard to manage the outside environment.

Alright, take a big breath; this list may seem daunting! The first stage is awareness and knowledge. Work your way down the list, concentrating on the exposures you believe to be most likely in your life. Fertility and general well-being can improve with small adjustments!

Your lifestyle has a direct impact on your capacity to conceive.

Avoid smoking. The use of tobacco is linked to decreased fertility. Smoking causes early egg depletion and ovarian aging. If you smoke, consult your medical professional for assistance in quitting.

Keep your alcohol consumption to a minimum. Ovulation problems are linked to a higher risk of heavy drinking. If you want to become pregnant, you might want to abstain from alcohol entirely. Since a safe amount of alcohol intake during fetal development has not been proven, abstinence at conception and during pregnancy is typically advised.

Reduce your caffeine intake. When used in moderation (less than 200 mg/day), caffeine does not appear to have an impact on female fertility. One or two 6- to 8-ounce cups of coffee per day should be the maximum amount of caffeine you consume.

Take care not to overtrain. Excessive levels of intense exercise can suppress progesterone production and prevent conception. If you are thinking about getting pregnant soon and you are at a healthy weight, you might want to restrict your intense exercise to no more than five hours per week.

Steer clear of toxic environments. Fertility can be negatively impacted by environmental contaminants and poisons, including lead, dry cleaning solvents, and pesticides

Nutrition

Your fertility may be significantly impacted by your diet. Eating a nutritious, well-balanced diet rich in whole grains, nuts, lean protein, and fresh produce is essential.

Your chances of conceiving naturally may be harmed by dietary decisions that result in weight gain or obesity, such as consuming an excessive amount of processed food.

Your hormone levels may be impacted by a bad diet, which might lead to irregular periods or issues with ovulation.

Mass (weight)

Both being underweight and being overweight might have an impact on fertility. It might be challenging for your body to ovulate and generate eggs if you are overweight. An additional factor contributing to ovulation and egg production issues is underweight.

See your doctor regarding your weight if you are attempting to conceive but have not been successful thus far. To increase your chances of becoming pregnant, they could advise you to gain or reduce weight.

Slumber

One of the most significant variables that might impact fertility is sleep.

Your ability to conceive may be significantly impacted by both the quantity and quality of your sleep.

Getting adequate sleep is essential for keeping the body and mind in good working order. Hormone balance is aided, which is necessary for both ovulation and pregnancy.

Make sure you set aside time each day for some sleep because not getting enough sleep at night may harm your capacity to conceive.

Chapter 3

What exactly are irregular periods?

Most women and persons designated female at birth have four to seven-day menstrual cycles. Your period occurs normally every 28 days, although regular menstrual cycles can last anywhere from 21 to 35 days. In actuality, the average length of a cycle is 29 days. Changes in hormone levels, stress, certain health problems, drugs, and other factors can contribute to irregular periods (or irregular menstruation).

What are some instances of erratic periods?

Your menstruation is still called "regular," even if it changes somewhat from cycle to cycle. Here are some examples of irregular menstruation:

• Intervals of less than 21 days or more than 35 days.

• Missing three or more consecutive periods.

• Significantly heavier or lower menstrual flow (bleeding) than normal.

• Periods lasting more than seven days .

• The time interval between cycles varies by more than nine days. For example, one cycle may last 28 days, another 37 days, and still another 29 days.

• Periods marked by extreme pain, cramps, nausea, or vomiting.

• Bleeding or spotting that occurs between periods, during menopause, or following sexual contact.

• Using one or more tampons or sanitary pads in one hour. Your menstrual cycle might not always be predictable, and that's okay. It is typical to see modest fluctuations in cycle duration or a menstrual period that appears somewhat heavier or lighter in flow than your prior period. Menstrual abnormalities are pretty frequent, and you don't have to be able to anticipate your period to the day to consider it "normal." Conditions associated with infrequent menstruation.

"Amenorrhea is a condition In which your periods have fully ceased. Unless you're pregnant, nursing, or going through menopause (which typically happens between the ages of 45 and 55), missing your period for 90 days or more is considered odd. If you haven't begun menstruation by the age of 15 or 16, or within three years of the development of your breasts, you may have amenorrhea. Oligomenorrhea is a condition in which your periods are irregular. You can have more than 35 days between periods or six to eight periods every year. Dysmenorrhea is a medical term for unpleasant menstrual cycles and severe cramping. It is common to have some discomfort during your period. Bleeding between monthly cycles, extended bleeding, or abnormally heavy menstruation are all examples of abnormal uterine bleeding.

What's causing my erratic periods?

Period irregularities can be caused by a variety of factors, ranging from stress to more serious underlying medical issues. Medical problems and irregular periods Missed menstrual cycles are related to certain health issues.

They are as follows:

- **Endometriosis.** occurs when endometrial tissue develops outside of the uterus. The tissue frequently adheres to your ovaries or fallopian tubes. Endometriosis can cause irregular bleeding, cramping, and severe discomfort before and during your period.

- **Pelvic inflammatory disease** (PID) PID is a bacterial illness that affects the female reproductive system. It is usually the result of an untreated sexually transmitted infection

(STI). Bacteria enter the vaginal cavity and spread to the uterus and upper genital tract. A thick vaginal discharge with an unpleasant odor, irregular periods, and pelvic discomfort are all symptoms of PID.

- **Polycystic ovarian syndrome** (PCOS) occurs when your ovaries produce an excessive quantity of androgens, a kind of hormone. This hormone suppresses or delays ovulation, resulting in irregular menstrual cycles. PCOS patients may experience a total cessation of menstruation.

- **Primary ovarian insufficiency:** This ailment affects cisgender women under the age of 40 whose ovaries do not function properly, resulting in missing or irregular periods. It can happen during cancer treatment with chemotherapy and radiation, or if you have a thyroid or pituitary gland disorder. Hormones are affected by hypothyroidism (underactive thyroid), hyperthyroidism (overactive thyroid), and other thyroid or pituitary gland illnesses. As a result, your menstruation will be erratic.

Chapter 4

Primary ovarian insufficiency is diagnosed.

What precisely is primary ovarian insufficiency?

Primary ovarian insufficiency, also known as primary ovarian failure, is an uncommon illness in which your ovaries cease to function before the age of 40. It causes irregular menstrual cycles and frequently results in infertility. The most prevalent treatment is hormone therapy (HT).

Primary ovarian insufficiency (POI) is a disorder in which the ovaries fail sooner than usual. During ovulation, your ovaries are tiny glands located on both sides of your uterus that manufacture and release eggs. Your ovaries also produce hormones that are necessary for menstruation, pregnancy, and other biological activities. Menopause, or the cessation of egg production, usually occurs at the age of 51. Some patients have POI unexpectedly, and they cease having a normal menstrual cycle. Others, on the other hand, are diagnosed with POI after months or years of irregular periods.

Premature ovarian failure was originally termed primary ovarian insufficiency. Healthcare practitioners, on the other hand, prefer the word "insufficiency" rather than "failure" because research has shown that patients with POI can experience sporadic ovulation. If you have POI, you can still release an egg and become pregnant. In reality, 5% to 10% of people with POI will become pregnant on their own without the need for infertility therapy. As a result, POI is also known as "decreased ovarian reserve."

What is the prevalence of primary ovarian insufficiency?

POI is uncommon, affecting around 1% of women or persons designated female at birth (AFAB) between the ages of 15 and 44. It can impact both people who have had children and those who have not. It is more frequent in adults over the age of 30.

What effects can primary ovarian insufficiency have on my body?

Low estrogen levels are caused by primary ovarian insufficiency. Loss of estrogen can cause symptoms comparable to menopause, such as hot flashes, reduced sex drive, and mood changes. It also raises your chances of developing osteoporosis, heart disease, and other diseases. Infertility is common in persons with primary ovarian insufficiency. Your provider, on the other hand, may be able to assist you in becoming pregnant through procedures such as the donation of eggs, IVF (in vitro fertilization), and/or fertility drugs.

What is the root cause of primary ovarian insufficiency?

The majority of the time, doctors do not know what causes primary ovarian insufficiency (idiopathic POI). However, evidence suggests that up to one-third of cases may be genetic.

Other reasons for POI include:

Autoimmune diseases such as Addison's disease, rheumatoid arthritis, and thyroid illness are examples of autoimmune disorders.

Chemotherapy and radiation therapy are two cancer therapies.

Turner syndrome (a genetic condition involving an anomaly in one of a person's AFAB's two X chromosomes) and Fragile X syndrome (a genetic disorder involving alterations in the gene FMR1) are examples of genetic disorders.

Hysterectomy (removal of the uterus).

Mumps and HIV are two examples of infections. (This is supposed to occur as a result of antibodies attacking your ovary.)

Prolonged contact with chemicals, insecticides, tobacco smoke, and other pollutants.

What are the symptoms and indicators of POI?

POI is most commonly manifested by irregular or skipped periods. Some women with primary ovarian insufficiency have no symptoms at all.

Other signs and symptoms may include:

- Period irregularity or absence.

Having difficulty becoming pregnant.

Reduced sexual urge.

- Concentration problems.

Irritability.

- Dry eyes.
- Tests and Diagnosis

How can you know if you have primary ovarian insufficiency?

A physical checkup and a pelvic exam will be performed by your healthcare practitioner. They will also inquire about your medical history. Knowing your regular menstrual cycle, prior pregnancies, and birth control use might assist your physician in diagnosing POI.

They will then most likely request blood tests to determine the levels of specific hormones in your body. FSH, estrogen, and prolactin are examples of these hormones.

Other tests that your provider may do include:

- A blood test to search for genetic problems (karyotype testing).
- A pelvic ultrasound will be performed to examine your ovaries and uterus.
- A pregnancy test.

How is primary ovarian insufficiency treated

POI is handled differently by different healthcare providers. It is determined by your age, symptoms, and desire to become pregnant. Treatment for primary ovarian insufficiency entails:

Taking the place of hormones that your ovaries no longer generate.

Treating POI symptoms or side effects (such as night sweats, vaginal dryness.

Lowering your risk of Poi-related disorders

HRT stands for hormone replacement treatment.

Hormone treatment provides your body with hormones that your ovaries do not produce. Hormone treatment may consist of taking just estrogen or estrogen plus progesterone. POI symptoms like night sweats and vaginal dryness can be reduced with hormone treatment. It will help reduce your chances of osteoporosis and other illnesses caused by POI. Hormone treatment may be prescribed in a variety of forms, including tablets, cream, gel, patch, or vaginal ring. If you start HRT, you'll be taking it until the age when natural menopause usually occurs (about 51 to 52). Discuss the advantages and dangers of HRT with your provider to ensure that it is appropriate for you.

Is It possible to reverse primary ovarian insufficiency?

No, basic ovarian insufficiency cannot be reversed. Medical professionals can treat symptoms, side effects, and linked illnesses, but they cannot cure them.

Can your ovaries begin to function again?

Even after diagnosis, around 25% of persons with POI may experience ovulation at least once. There is, however, no therapy that can help your ovaries start working again. Treatment for primary ovarian insufficiency relieves symptoms and minimizes your chance of developing health problems caused by POI.

www.ingramcontent.com/pod-product-compliance
Lightning Source LLC
Chambersburg PA
CBHW070856260726
48661CB00004B/1436